Yoga: A Way of Life

A Beginner's Guide to Yoga as Much More Than Just a Fitness Routine

Sara Elliott price

Published in The USA by:

Success Life Publishing

125 Thomas Burke Dr.

Hillsborough, NC 27278

Copyright © 2015 by Sara Elliott Price

ISBN-10: 1511872640

Disclaimer

Every effort has been made to accurately represent this book and its potential. Results vary with every individual, and your results may or may not be different from those depicted. No promises, guarantees or warranties, whether stated or implied, have been made that you will produce any specific result from this book. Your efforts are individual and unique, and may vary from those shown. Your success depends on your efforts, background and motivation.

The material in this publication is provided for educational and informational purposes only and is not intended as medical advice. The information contained in this book should not be used to diagnose or treat any illness, metabolic disorder, disease or health problem. Always consult your physician or health care provider before beginning any nutrition or exercise program. Use of the programs, advice, and information contained in this book is at the sole choice and risk of the reader.

Table of Contents

Introduction...1

Chapter 1 - History of Yoga 3

Chapter 2 - Pranayama or Breath Control 9

Chapter 3 - Asanas or Postures 17

Chapter 4 - Other Practices of Hatha Yoga............................. 26

Chapter 5 - Three Yogas for Three Types of People.................30

Chapter 6 - Raja Yoga..38

Conclusion 43

Introduction

Yoga is immensely popular around the world today as a form of exercise. It is great for increasing flexibility, improving balance, strengthening the core and recovering from injuries. Meditation, mindfulness and breath control are also practiced with Yoga and it is considered a legitimate way of reducing stress. Some people are also aware of the spiritual benefits of practicing Yoga.

This Yoga that is popular in the Western world is but one school of Yoga called Hatha Yoga. There are a lot of other schools of Yoga but very few people understand Yoga in its entirety. Yoga is much more than exercise and meditation. At its essence it is a philosophy and a way of living life. The benefits of Yoga go beyond physical, mental and spiritual health. When understood properly and applied completely, Yoga can help you live "the good life."

Whether you are a complete novice at Yoga or a regular practitioner, this book will help you increase your understanding of Yoga. You'll read about the origins of Yoga and the various schools of Yoga that you can follow in your life.

In this book you'll learn about:

- The origins of Yoga.

- The five schools of Yoga.

- The common practices of Hatha Yoga.

- The practices of Raja Yoga.

- Jnana Yoga, Bhakti Yoga and Karma Yoga for three different types of people.

- The benefits of following Yoga as a way of life.

Consider this book but a primer on the real Yoga. Once you understand the different schools of Yoga, you'll naturally gravitate towards the areas that will help you the most. You can then apply these practices and learn more deeply about them to align your life with the philosophy of Yoga.

Chapter 1 - History of Yoga

Yoga originated in ancient India. The exact date of origin can not be confirmed but the most popular theory is that Yoga developed during the Vedic times around 6th century BCE. According to this theory the Vedic monks used certain postures and meditative practices while performing Yajna, a holy ceremony involving fire. These postures slowly evolved into the practice of Yoga.

The word Yoga has different meanings and can mean 'to join' or 'to yoke' as in joining the Atman or individual soul with the Brahman or universal soul. It can also mean 'to concentrate' or meditate.

With time Yoga merged with philosophy and developed into different schools. It also spread into other religions such as Jainism and Buddhism and even Islam. Yoga spread to the west in the 19th century and Swami Vivekananda was the one who made it popular along with other eastern philosophical concepts, among the intellectuals, spiritualists and transcendentalists of the west. In the last few decades, Yoga has grown in popularity throughout the world but mostly as a fitness regimen and as a method for relieving stress.

There are 5 main schools of Yoga that exist today.

1. Hatha Yoga:

Hatha Yoga primarily involves strengthening the body and achieving prime physical health. It includes two practices that are very popular today; Pranayama or breath control and Asanas or body postures. For most people these two practices are all there is to Yoga but actually these are just a part of Hatha Yoga. You'll see below that these practices are also a part of Raja Yoga which tries to include the best practices of all previous schools of Yoga.

There are two more practices in Hatha Yoga. One is called Shat Karmas or Six Purifications. These are practices to cleanse the internal organs such as the nasal tract and intestines etc. These are higher level practices of Hatha Yoga that can help in staying healthy by cleansing the body from within.

Laya Yoga is the fourth practice of Hatha Yoga which is also called Kundalini Awakening. This part of Hatha Yoga crosses the realm of physical fitness and talks about spiritual fitness. The concept of Kundalini and Chakras will be discussed in detail in a later chapter but for now know that it is a form of meditation that is used for awakening the spiritual energy within you.

4

2. Jnana Yoga:

Jnana means knowledge and this path of Yoga is for the intellectual types who need to understand things from a logical point of view. Eastern philosophy is sometimes considered irrational but Jnana Yoga encourages gaining logical knowledge of the world and your own self so that you can build the base to enter the spiritual realm.

The focus of this path is to move beyond literal knowledge and try to 'see' the truth without the need of 'understanding' it. By doing Jnana Yoga you can achieve the connection to the universal soul through the path of knowledge and wisdom.

3. Bhakti Yoga:

Bhakti means devotion or worship. This form of Yoga is for the emotional romantic who is devoted to God. The Vedic culture, out of which Hinduism developed, was a tolerant culture that encouraged all forms of thought even including atheism. When Bhakti Yoga talks about devotion to a God, it doesn't refer to a particular Hindu God but to a personal God that can vary from individual to individual.

This is why Yoga is truly a secular way of life because it doesn't try to force any particular religion on anyone. Whether you believe in a God of any religion, or even if you only have a faint idea of a Supreme Being or universal soul, you can use Bhakti Yoga to achieve the same connection with the divine through worship and devotion.

4. Karma Yoga:

Karma is a famous term around the world as the philosophy of cause and effect which states that you reap as you sow and sooner or later you receive the results of your Karma. So you should do good to earn good Karma so that in the future you get good results.

But Karma literally means action and Karma Yoga is the path of Yoga for the man of action. Unlike the intellectuals who would prefer Jnana Yoga and the romantics who'd choose Bhakti Yoga, Karma Yoga is for those who believe in doing. By living your normal life and doing all your actions without getting attached to their results, you can still achieve the union with the divine.

5. Raja Yoga:

Finally we have the fifth school of Yoga known as the Raja Yoga. Raja Yoga was formed much later and tried to include the best of every other form of Yoga. It talks about an eightfold path to achieve physical, mental and spiritual health that eventually leads to Moksha or Nirvana or enlightenment.

The eightfold path includes:

1. Yama or Five Abstentions

2. Niyama or Five Observances

3. Asanas or Eighty-four Balanced Postures

4. Pranayama or Breath Control

5. Pratyahara or Withdrawal of Senses

6. Dharana or Concentration

7. Dhyana or Meditation

8. Samadhi or Deep Meditation

We'll talk about all of these eight folds in a later chapter but as you can see Pranayama and Asanas are a part of this Yoga along with Dhyana or meditation. The Yoga that is practiced commonly today contains these three elements but since it is mostly related to physical fitness and stress release, we can say that it is part of Hatha Yoga which is concerned mostly with physical fitness.

Raja Yoga includes spiritual practices that help you in rising above emotional attachment and desires and achieve enlightenment. Apart from these 5 major schools of Yoga there are also different styles of Yoga that are popular today. Some of these styles are; Ananda Yoga, Ashtanga Yoga, Integral Yoga, Iyengar Yoga, Shivananda Yoga etc. These are usually just different versions of Hatha Yoga or Raja Yoga that have been made popular by a particular teacher of Yoga. For example Iyengar Yoga is a harder version of Hatha Yoga that was formulated by B.K.S Iyengar in the 70s.

For the current discussion we'll not go deeper into these varying styles of Yoga. In the coming chapters we'll talk about all the schools of Yoga and how to apply them in your life. Since Pranayama and Asanas are the most popular form of Yoga we'll explore these topics in more detail.

Chapter 2 - Pranayama or Breath Control

Pranayama is the practice of controlling your breath. It has spread around the world along with the body postures as part of Yoga meditation. But in reality Pranayama is much more than just breathe control.

Prana means 'life force' and it is a Vedic philosophical concept which says that everything in the universe is made of Prana. You might find it interesting to know that particle physicists are also coming to a similar conclusion that the smallest form of matter is nothing but a web of potential that exists in the entire universe and out of which matter and energy is formed.

According to the Vedas, by regulating our breath we can also regulate this vital energy or life force within us. This helps in attaining perfect physical, mental, emotional and spiritual health. Scientifically speaking, breathing deeply and rhythmically has been shown to have tremendous benefits.

Basic Deep Breathing

In the most basic form Pranayama is about breathing deeply. If you watch an infant breathe, you'll notice that its belly rises and falls with every breath. But as adults we forget deep breathing and only take short breaths, inflating just our chest.

This means that a large part of the lungs is not used in normal day to day breathing.

Scientifically speaking, it means that we only use about half of our lung capacity which leads to an oxygen deficiency in the body. With less oxygen, the body operates on a less than optimal level. Short breathing also means that the blood is not purified of all of its carbon dioxide. Low oxygen and CO_2 in the body together lead to low energy, lethargy, stress, inability to concentrate and perform tasks at our best level. It also leads to exhaustion and reduction in the life of our body cells.

In other words by breathing shallow and short breaths, we underperform and age faster. This is why deep breathing, not just as a once-a-day practice but also as something to be aware of throughout the day, can help us improve our physical and mental health.

You can start by practicing deep breathing once or twice a day and then try to use it throughout the day whenever you realize that you've been breathing shallow. To do this, sit in a comfortable position and put your hand on your belly. Inhale slowly and feel your stomach inflate with air. Hold the breath for a short while and let the blood extract all the oxygen from the lungs. Exhale slowly till your stomach contracts inwards. Repeat a few times and try to breathe this way throughout the day.

You can also practice deep breathing if you are feeling anxious or nervous or stressed out about something. When we are tense our breathing slows down and just by consciously changing our breathing pattern we can control our heart rate and come out of the tense feeling.

In Pranayama there are a lot of different breathing techniques that go beyond this simple deep breathing. A few major techniques of Pranayama are:

Anulom Vilom

Anulom Vilom Pranayama is also called the Nadi Shuddhi Pranayama. To practice Anulom Vilom technique of Pranayama you need to follow the following steps:

1. Sit in a comfortable position, preferably cross legged on the ground. If you can comfortably do it, sit in the lotus position; cross legged with both feet coming up and resting on the opposite thighs. If this is too hard you can try the half lotus position in which only one foot comes up and other is below the thigh. Or use the normal cross legged position with both feet below the thighs. Your back and neck should be straight but not rigid. If you have knee or back problems you can also sit on a chair with your back straight, knees together and both feet touching the floor.

2. Place your left hand over your left knee, palm facing upwards and the index finger curled and touching the thumb.

3. Fold the index and ring fingers of your right hand while the thumb and remaining two fingers are outstretched. Place the right hand over your mouth so that the two curled fingers are resting on the lips.

4. Close your right nostril by pressing it with the thumb and inhale from the left nostril. Hold the breath and close the left nostril with the last two fingers. Open the right nostril and exhale.

5. Repeat the same process but this time starting with the right nostril which is now open while the left is closed. Inhale from the right and then close the right nostril and open the left to exhale.

6. Repeat this cycle for 5 to 10 minutes.

By practicing this technique you can cleanse the two nerves which are said to control the mental force and the vital life force. By achieving a balance between the two, you can awaken the spiritual cord or the Kundalini.

Anulom Vilom can also help you improve blood circulation, relax the body and mind, improve concentration, relieve stress, depression and hypertension.

Kapalbhati

Kapalbhati is a technique that is great for relieving stomach problems such as acidity, constipation etc. and it can also help in weight loss. Here's a step by step procedure to do Kapalbhati:

1. Sit cross legged as for Anulom Vilom. You can't sit in a chair for this one as it involves exercising the abdominal muscles. But if you have problem sitting cross legged you can try the Thunderbolt Pose in which you kneel and rest your thighs on your calves.

2. Keep the eyes closed and place the hands on your knees with the palm facing up and the index finger touching the thumb.

3. Inhale normally and then exhale with all your force so that your stomach goes all the way in. The purpose is to exhale by pulling in your stomach as hard as you can.

4. Exhale through both nostrils. Explosive expulsion of the air should produce a hissing sound.

5. Don't think too much about inhaling and let it remain on autopilot. You don't need to inhale deeply for this technique. Just focus on exhaling.

6. Do one exhalation per second and repeat for 5 minutes. Rest for a minute and then do another 5 minute cycle. You can do this technique for up to 30 minutes.

Ujjayi

Ujjayi is also known as Ocean breath for the sound that is produced during this technique, although literally it translates to Victorious Breath. To perform this technique, follow these steps:

1. Sit in a cross legged position as in Anulom Vilom. You can sit on a chair for this one if needed.

2. Keep your hands on your knees as mentioned earlier and your spine straight.

3. Inhale through both nostrils but narrow the throat passage to constrict the airway. This will lead to a long drawn out breath and also produce a hissing sound.

4. Exhale through the nose with the throat passage still constricted to produce a similar sound.

5. Balance the inhalation and exhalation so that both last the same amount of time. Repeat for 5 to 10 minutes.

Ujjayi technique will strengthen your diaphragm and increase your lung capacity. It is also good for throat related problems such as thyroid gland problems etc. It is also said to provide vital energy to the body so that you can perform hard physical tasks with ease. This is why it is sometimes performed before practicing the Asanas or postures to improve physical performance.

Bhramari

Bhramari Pranayama is known as the Humming Bee Pranayama because you make a humming sound that resembles the buzz of a bee. Follow the following steps to perform this technique:

1. Sit in a comfortable position like for the rest of the techniques.

2. Place the thumbs of both hands over the ear canal, blocking the ears. The index fingers are placed just above the eyebrows on the forehead while the middle fingers close the eyes.

3. Inhale deeply and slowly through the nose.

4. Exhale slowly through both nostrils while making a humming sound.

5. Repeat for 3 to 5 minutes.

Bhramari is good for releasing tension, anger, anxiety and frustration. It also cures sinus problems and high blood pressure.

These are just 4 of over 50 techniques of Pranayama. It is suggested to practice these techniques after learning from an experienced teacher, as some of these can cause harm if not done properly. Since Prana is the vital life force, you have to be careful about correct technique while doing Pranayama.

Chapter 3 - Asanas or Postures

The most famous part of Yoga is the Asanas or postures that are meant to improve physical fitness by improving flexibility, balance and muscle strength. Yoga postures also improve overall health by keeping the internal organs performing at their optimum level.

As mentioned earlier, there are several techniques named after particular teachers who gave their own spin to the postures. Some like Iyengar Yoga have a high level of difficulty and are meant for experienced practitioners, while others like Ananda Yoga can be performed even by the most inexperienced beginners.

Choosing which technique of Yoga postures to use depends on your fitness level and your ultimate goal with Yoga. But here in this book I'd like to introduce you to the most basic form of Asanas.

In total there are 84 different postures, each one focusing on a different set of body parts. Covering all of the poses is beyond the scope of this book as some of the postures are for experienced practitioners only. Instead I'll introduce the postures to you through 8 of the most basic Asanas.

1. Padmasana (Lotus Pose)

The most basic Asana of all is the Padmasana or the Lotus Pose, so called because the foot lock position resembles the petals of a lotus flower. This is the same posture that I talked about in the last chapter on Pranayama. It is used for both Pranayama and meditation.

To perform this Asana, sit on a mat or soft but thin cushion with both legs stretched out in front of you. Bend the right knee and bring the right foot over the left thigh with the sole facing upwards and the heel pressing in the groin. Now bend the left knee and place the left foot on the right thigh with the sole facing upwards. Both knees should touch the ground. The spine should maintain its normal curvature. The chest should be thrust slightly forwards and the shoulders moved back. Lower the chin towards the neck so as to align the neck with the spine. Both hands should be resting on respective knees with the palm facing upwards and the index finger touching the thumb.

This Asana can be done on its own for a few minutes or used to perform meditation or Pranayama. When you sit in this posture the large amount of blood that flows into your legs is redirected to the abdomen and the organs in that area benefit with this increased flow. This posture also provides balance and stability and allows you to sit steadily for long periods of time so that you can focus your mind on meditation. By holding the spine in the natural position it helps in unobstructed flow of Prana or vital energy through the entire body and also helps in raising the Kundalini energy.

2. Vajrasana (Thunderbolt Pose)

Vajrasana is the second sitting pose that can be used for Pranayama especially Kapalbhati. It is known as the Thunderbolt Pose as 'Vajra' translates to thunderbolt but the body is not shaped like a thunderbolt in this asana. Instead its name is derived from the fact that it affects a nerve called the Vajra Nadi. It is also sometimes called the diamond pose or the adamantine pose.

To do this Asana, you need to sit on the floor or on a mat with your knees touching the ground. The right toe should be placed over the left two as the soles of both your feet face upwards. The soles of the feet will form a semicircular 'cushion' on which you will rest your buttocks. Your legs from toe to knee should be touching the floor. Both the thighs will rest on the respective calves. You can place your hands on your knees, palm facing down. Keep the spine straight and the neck, head and trunk should be in one line.

You should hold this Asana for 5-10 minutes. This is the only Asana that you can do even after having a meal. It helps in aiding digestion and relives problems such as constipation, flatulence, indigestion etc.

3. Sarvangasana (All-Member Pose)

Sarva means whole and Anga means limb or body part. So Sarvangasana is the Asana for the entire body. It is also known as Shoulder-stand and is known as the mother of all Asanas.

To perform this Asana you start by lying on the floor with your legs straight and the arms on both sides with palms facing downwards. Raise the legs so that they are perpendicular to the floor. Then move the legs towards your head by lifting the torso off the floor. Once your feet are touching the floor behind your head you are in a pose known as Halasana. From here raise your legs and torso so that your entire weight is on the shoulders. Bend your arms at the elbows to support your torso. Your chest should be pushed into the chin. The back of the head and the neck should be flat on the floor.

The legs and torso should be in line and at 90 degrees from the floor. Your toes should be stretched out and inline with the eyes. Hold this pose without shaking or swaying for as long as possible. Breathe normally but do no swallow while you are in the inverted pose.

This Asana exercises the entire body and effects all the glands and organs of the body but has the most effect on the thyroid gland located in the neck. Do not attempt this Asana if you have back or neck problems, arthritis, osteoporosis, high blood pressure and during menstruation. This Asana should also be followed immediately by Matsyasana.

4. Matsyasana (Fish Pose)

Matsyasana or fish pose is good for stretching the spine and cervical region and that's why it is combined with Sarvangasana. It opens up the chest and helps in deep breathing. It can cure diseases of the respiratory system such as asthma and chronic bronchitis. It can also help in relieving constipation as the abdominal region experiences pressure during the pose.

To perform this pose you need to be sitting in Padmasana. Bend backwards and lie flat on your back. Your hands should be on your sides with the palms facing downwards. Now bend your back by raising your torso off the ground by pushing down on your elbows and forearms. Let the head hang back but it should not touch the floor. This is the basic Matsyasana but you can take it one step further by grabbing the big toe of both feet by your hands and pulling the feet inwards. This will help in arching the back even more and your chest will open up further.

This Asana strengthens the muscles of the neck, back and the abdomen.

5. Dhanurasana (Bow Pose)

Dhanurasana resembles a bow where the hands form the string and the body forms the bow.

To perform Dhanurasana lie flat on your stomach on the floor. Your arms should be on your sides. Bend the knees and bring the feet up to the buttocks. Grab each foot with the respective hand keeping all fingers and the thumb on the outside of the foot. Now stretch your legs so that your chest and thighs rise off the floor. Your body should be balanced on your abdomen. You can also induce a seesaw motion backwards and forwards and then sideways to massage the abdomen muscles.

This Asana is great for relieving problems of the gastro-intestinal tract such as constipation, indigestion and dyspepsia. It improves liver function and also makes the spine more elastic. It also helps with rheumatism of the legs, hands and knees. It also reduces fat and tones the abdomen.

6. Pashchimottana Asana (Posterior Stretching Pose)

Despite it's hard to pronounce name, Pashchimottana Asana is performed even by those who don't do Yoga. Athletes use this to stretch their hamstrings and back.

To perform this Asana you need to be sitting on the floor with your legs stretched straight in front of you. The knees and feet should be touching each other. Raise your arms up above your head so that they are touching your ears and perpendicular to the floor. Now bend forwards from the waist and bring your arms down to touch your feet. At advanced level you should be able to grip the soles of your feet and touch your head to your knees but in the beginning stretch as much as you can.

This is one Asana in which you don't need to hold the pose for too long and instead you should go back to the perpendicular position and then repeat the stretch several times.

As mentioned earlier it is great for stretching hamstrings and the muscles of the buttocks and lower back. It also keeps the spine elastic and helps in relieving disorders related to digestion, liver problems, diabetes etc.

7. Chakra Asana (Wheel Pose)

Chakra means a wheel or a circle. This is a backbend pose in which your spine is stretched and loosened and the entire body becomes more flexible and energized.

To perform this Asana you need to lie on the ground on your back with your arms on your side. Now bend the knees and bring your feet close to your buttocks. They should be one foot or shoulder length apart. Now bring your hands to the sides of your head so that the palms are touching the floor with the fingers towards your shoulders. Now push up and raise your entire body so that you form a circular shape and your body is stabilized on your feet and hands. Make sure your head is hanging loose and the neck is not stiff.

8. Bakasana (Crane Pose)

The final Asana I'm going to talk about here is the Crane Pose or Bakasana. It is also sometimes called the Crow Pose.

To perform this Asana crouch on the floor with your feet close together. Place your hands shoulder width apart in front of you with the fingers facing forwards. This position should resemble a frog. Now tilt slightly forwards and lift the feet off the ground. Rest your shins on the backside of the upper arms just above the elbows. You should be balanced on your hands and your arms should be as straight as possible. Hold this pose for up to 2 minutes.

It might not be possible to achieve stable balance in the beginning but with practice you will be able to do it with ease. This pose will strengthen your arms, chest, shoulders and core. It will improve balance and overall strength.

These 8 Asanas should get you off with the postures part of Yoga. There is no dearth of teachers when it comes to postures as this is what Yoga is considered to be all about and you should be able to find good teachers to teach you the rest of the advanced Asanas when you are ready to move to the higher levels. But as I've mentioned this is just a part of Yoga. In the next chapter we'll talk about the other two remaining practices of Hatha Yoga.

Chapter 4 - Other Practices of Hatha Yoga

Apart from Pranayama and Asanas, there are two more practices in Hatha Yoga that take care of the overall physical health and well being of the Yogi.

Shat Karmas or Six Purifications

These are practices that cleanse the body of all its impurities. This is a high level of Yoga that should not be practiced without the guidance of a teacher. The six purifications are:

1. **Neti**: This can be done using warm water or a soft thread. The thread is inserted in one nostril and taken out of the mouth and then repeated through the other nostril. It cleanses the nasal passages.

2. **Dhoti**: A soft thing piece of cloth, about 3 inches wide and 12 feet long is swallowed till the tip is left in the mouth and then taken back out. The food canal and stomach is cleansed through this practice.

3. **Basti**: This is a form of enema in which you sit in a tub full of water and water is drawn into the intestines through the anus and then expelled. This cleanses the colon.

4. **Nyoli**: In this practice the muscles of the abdomen are used to churn the stomach and intestines from side to side. This strengthens the intestines and relieves constipation.

5. **Bhasrika**: This means to breath through each nostril with a lot of force like a bellow. This is usually done after Neti and it too helps in cleaning the nasal passages.

6. **Trataka**: In this practice you have to focus at the junction of the eyebrows and stare at it without blinking till the eyes start to water. This improves eyesight.

These practices might seem extreme to the beginner but these have been practiced by experienced Yogis for centuries and are proven to be of immense benefit.

Kundalini Awakening or Laya Yoga

Kundalini Awakening is a concept that is popular in the western world and has been adopted into several similar systems. Kundalini Yoga is even considered to be a free standing concept with Pranayama and Asanas being a part of it. But here I'll talk about the original concept of Kundalini as a part of Hatha Yoga.

Kundalini is a spiritual energy that is said to be lying dormant in most people at the base of the spine in a coil. The word

Kundalini comes from 'Kundali' which means the coil of a snake. The purpose of the Yogi is to awaken this energy and make it rise through the Chakras in the body. It is also called as Laya Yoga because 'Laya' means extinguishing or disappearance and means the disappearance of the faults of the ego as the Kundalini rises through each Chakra In the end the Kundalini can merge with the universal energy and result in the disappearance of duality so that the person can experience the ultimate reality first hand.

The major Chakras through which the Kundalini rises are:

1. Muladhara Chakra or Root Chakra located at the base of the spine.

2. Svadhishthana Chakra or Sacral Chakra located slightly above the pelvis near the generative organs.

3. Manipura Chakra or Navel Chakra located at the navel.

4. Anahata Chakra or Heart Chakra located at the level of the nipples in the chest.

5. Vishuddha Chakra or Throat Chakra located behind the vocal chords.

6. Ajna Chakra or Third-eye Chakra located at the point where the eyebrow lines meet above the nose.

7. Sahasrara Chakra or Crown Chakra located slightly above the crown of the head.

Each Chakra is related to certain emotions and states of being and the Kundalini rising through the Chakras represents the spiritual journey of the Yogi.

As per Hatha Yoga, in order to awaken your Kundalini you need to meditate and focus on the different Chakras and will your Kundalini to awaken and rise. Alongside you also need to be practicing all the rest of Hatha Yoga as everything is interconnected and as you move to higher levels of Yoga your Kundalini will automatically rise through the appropriate Chakras.

All this talk about Kundalini energy might not seem too scientific to some but it is based on the practical experience of Yogis from thousands of years ago. You don't need to believe in any of it but as long as you practice Pranayama and Asanas, your Kundalini will begin to rise. In the next chapter we'll talk about some other schools of Yoga.

Chapter 5 - Three Yogas for Three Types of People

As described in the Vedas, you can practice Yoga through the daily work of your life as well. For this there are three schools of Yoga for three types of individuals. But it should be noted that only rarely will one person fit completely into one stereotype and most of us can use some parts of all three of these paths.

1. Jnana Yoga

If you are an intellectual, a man of thought, someone who likes to think through problems till you come to a logical solution, then Jnana Yoga is for you. Jnana means knowledge and this is the path on which you can seek enlightenment through knowledge.

It is significant that Yoga has such a path because most people think that all eastern philosophy is irrational and mystical. The truth is that in Yoga there is a path for everyone. Psychologists believe that if a person can become consciously aware about the root cause of their neurosis then they can overcome it. In a similar way Jnana Yoga says that by understanding the true nature of reality one can reach enlightenment.

In order to walk on this spiritual path of knowledge you need to answer the question of who you really are. Are you the physical body or the mind or both? Or are you the consciousness that arises out of this body and the electrochemical processes of the brain?

To practice Jnana Yoga you need to take the following steps:

- End ignorance as ignorance is the cause of all suffering. When we stay ignorant about the true nature of the world and our own true nature, we stay stuck in the world of emotions and desires which lead to a constant cycle of happiness and suffering. And as we all know the suffering seems to be much more than the happiness. You can break this cycle by studying about the true nature of the world and your own self.

- Know that you are not the body. The body is just a vehicle used by the consciousness which is the real you. You need to become aware of how your ego leads to your identification with your body and your image in the society. When you are attached to your ego, you are a slave to your emotions. Anything that hurts your ego will cause you suffering because you think that's you. But in reality you are not the ego, you are the consciousness which is a part of the universal consciousness, just like every other human being and in fact all life on earth.

- Understand that the material world is just an illusion created by us. This world where we have created borders and divisions of caste, color, race and creed, is not real. In reality we are all manifestations of the same universal consciousness.

- By understanding these truths you can develop a peaceful state of mind that does not suffer from a lot of anxiety, frustration and stress.

- Control your emotions, desires, urges and the needs of the body by using all of this knowledge. Rise above physical discomfort and pleasure and pain.

- Be content with what you have and where you are. This state of mind can only come after you've spent a lot of time contemplating the true nature of yourself and the world.

- Develop a strong character that allows you to endure all hardships of life without getting hopeless or frustrated. Have faith in the knowledge that no matter how bad things get, it's just another experience for the real you which is your consciousness.

In this way the path of knowledge can lead to spiritual enlightenment.

2. Bhakti Yoga

If Jnana Yoga didn't connect with you then maybe you are an emotional and romantic person who values gut feeling over logical conclusions. For such a person there is the path of devotion or Bhakti Yoga.

This path might not be all that popular today as religion has got a bad reputation over the years and more and more people are choosing to be atheists or agnostics. But if you do believe in a god, complete devotion to that god can also lead to spiritual enlightenment. It doesn't matter which god you believe in as Yoga doesn't try to force any religion on you. What does matter is the nature of the devotion. It has to be complete devotion and unshakable faith that is required on the path of Bhakti Yoga.

In practice Bhakti Yogis spend a lot of time praying, singing devotional songs and worshiping their personal god in any way. But it doesn't always have to be that way. As long as you devote your entire life and direct all your actions according to the will of god, you can be on the path of Bhakti Yoga even while living a normal life.

It is important to mention that the path of Bhakti Yoga can be considered controversial, especially in today's environment. If Bhakti Yoga means blind faith in your god and doing whatever your god wills then is a terrorist suicide bomber who kills innocents and commits suicide just to please a god, a Bhakti Yogi? We know that in reality it is not the will of any god to slaughter innocents of other religion. It is only how the name of god is used, and his message distorted by power hungry priests, that leads to such horrifying acts.

But how does one differentiate the word of some priest or holy man from the true will of god? Bhakti Yoga says that in order to do this you need to let your love for your god be the guide to the truth. If you let your instincts and emotions guide you, you won't be easily driven astray by any one trying to abuse the god's name for personal gain.

Bhakti Yoga shows that if the path of devotion and love towards a personal god appeals to you, you can use it to achieve spiritual enlightenment.

3. Karma Yoga

For those who believe in action rather than in philosophy or devotion, there is the path of the Karma Yoga. As mentioned earlier Karma basically means action. The law of Karma that is popular worldwide says that for every action you get an equivalent spiritual reaction. So if you do good deeds, you'll get good results and if you do bad deeds you'll get bad results.

Karma Yoga says that there is also a third option. If you do disinterested action you will break free of the cycle of Karma and won't get any reaction, good or bad. This is what a Karma Yogi should try to achieve in their daily life.

Disinterested action means to do action without getting attached to the results of our action. When we do anything, we do it to achieve a particular goal. Every action is aligned with a goal. So if you study for an exam you are doing so because you want to do well in it. There is nothing wrong with having goals but it is the attachment to these goals that causes suffering.

So if you are attached to the idea of scoring high in the exam and you start dreaming about how proud your family, teachers and friends are going to be then you've become attached to a particular result. This means that if you don't achieve a favorable result you will suffer the pain of failure. Not only that, but once you get attached to scoring high, you build up unnecessary pressure on yourself which makes you suffer through every day before the exam. Ironically, this pressure might actually hinder your performance and lead to failure.

According to Karma Yoga, in this situation, you should just study for the sake of studying and stop thinking about the results. The idea is to not get attached to a particular result. Your aim should be to study well right now and that's it.

Whether you score high or not should not bother you. There can be conditions outside your control that might lead to your scoring less. For example if the scores will be a percentile, you might do really well but still not score in the high percentile because a lot of other students did better than you.

In life there are even more complex situations and we make the mistake of getting attached to the results of our actions and when they don't turn out the way we thought they should, we get disappointed. Over the years this leads to a negative attitude that makes it impossible to achieve anything because we get attached to the result and from the beginning start telling ourselves that we'll fail at it and we imagine the humiliation of failure and put unnecessary pressure on ourselves.

Disinterested action is the way out of this vicious cycle. To perform disinterested action means to do things for the sake of doing them. There is an enjoyment in getting completely focused and doing any activity for a while and that alone should be the goal of a Karma Yogi.

When you combine practices of Hatha Yoga for physical and mental health and lead a life that is ruled by some combination of Jnana, Bhakti and Karma Yoga, you can truly live a wonderful life that will not only help you grow spiritually but also make every day full of peace and bliss. This is the idea of Raja Yoga which we'll talk about in the next chapter.

Chapter 6 - Raja Yoga

So far we've learned about Hatha Yoga which is primarily for gaining physical health, and we've learned three philosophical schools of Yoga; Jnana, Bhakti and Karma, that tell us how we should live our life. To combine all this we have the final school of Yoga known as Raja Yoga. You can translate Raja Yoga as the King of all Yogas. It includes the best of all previous schools.

Raja Yoga was expounded by a Hindu Yogi known as Patanjali. The many different modern schools of Yoga are based on this original school. It is also known as the Ashtanga Yoga because Ashtanga translates as 'eight limbs' which correspond to the eightfold path taught by this Yoga.

Raja Yoga says that people suffer from five afflictions or problems that cause them to stay stuck in the world of ego and desires and causes all of their suffering. **The 5 afflictions are:**

1. Avidya or Ignorance

2. Asmita or Ego

3. Raga or Desire

4. Dvesha or Aversion

5. Abhinivesha or The Attachment to Life

Ignorance, as mentioned earlier is about taking the illusory world to be real and staying stuck in it. Ego or I-ness is the misidentification with this body and mind as the real you. The ego results in the creation of this illusory world and ignorance keeps us stuck in it.

Desires and aversions are two sides of the same coin. Desire means to seek pleasure and aversion means to seek the avoidance of pain. Both of these lead to suffering because we can't fulfill all our desires and we can't avoid all pain in life.

The attachment to life is the desire to continue living. It can also be called as the fear of death. We live our lives ignoring our own immortality because we don't want to face death. Combine this with desires, aversions, ego and ignorance and we end up living an automatic life that is out of our control and we are just reacting to our surroundings and the people around us.

By removing all these afflictions we can lead a peaceful and meaningful life. This does not equate to a life that has no suffering and only happiness. There will still be the natural cycles of sorrow and joy but we can find a way to stay peaceful despite all the fluctuations in our emotions.

Removing ignorance is the first step to becoming aware of all this. Letting go of the ego can lead to a simplification of life. If we don't try to fulfill our desires we can end half of our suffering and we can learn to accept the rest of the suffering by letting go of our aversions. Finally by accepting the fact that we will eventually die, we can live a more meaningful life.

To cure us of all these aversions, Raja Yoga offers an eightfold path.

1. Yama or Five Abstentions

2. Niyama or Five Observances

3. Asanas or Postures

4. Pranayama or Breath Control

5. Pratyahara or Withdrawal of Senses

6. Dharana or Concentration

7. Dhyana or Meditation

8. Samadhi or Deep Meditation

Yama and Niyama together form the ten commandments of Raja Yoga. According to these you should abstain from violence, lying, stealing, sensuality and greed. And you should observe purity of body and mind, contentment, self discipline, studiousness and resignation to god. The last one means to leave the results to fate or god and only concern yourself with disinterested action.

The next two steps are the postures and breath control that we talked about in Hatha Yoga.

The fifth step is withdrawal of senses. This means to learn to control your senses in such a way that you become their master and no sensation can ruin your concentration. This is achieved by withdrawing senses from the sense objects. One example is that Raja Yogi's won't eat for the sake of taste. Their food is functional and bland and this helps in controlling the sense of taste. By controlling all the senses in this way we can develop a high level of concentration which is the sixth step.

Concentration leads to improved meditation. During meditation the Yogi can go beyond concentrating on the breath or on a particular point. Meditation is the state when you are completely present in the moment. Samadhi or deep meditation is the highest level of meditation in which you become one with the universe. You lose all sense of your ego and stop identifying with your body and mind. Instead you become the universe and your consciousness merges with the universal consciousness.

Samadhi is the ultimate aim of Raja Yoga and can only be achieved after years of practicing the first seven steps of the eightfold path. In this way Raja Yoga provides a step by step process to become a true Yogi. As you can see, it is much more than just Pranayama and Asanas and includes philosophy, spirituality and a complete way of living life.

Conclusion

In the end I just want to say that if you liked this book, your journey as a Yogi has only begun. This book only gives a thorough introduction to what Yoga truly is. It tries to make you aware of Yoga as much more than just a way to get fit and relieve stress.

The benefits of body postures will be yours even if you don't follow anything else but if you do choose to adopt the philosophy of Yoga in your life, I can assure you that you'll gain many more benefits than just improved health and fitness.

If you are wondering where to go from here, just begin with the parts of Yoga that speak to you. Maybe you aren't convinced about the spiritual benefits of Yoga and only want to do it for fitness. Maybe you liked the philosophy of Karma Yoga and want to adopt it along with the body postures. You can do whatever you want. Start with whatever parts speak to you and explore others only if you feel inclined towards them.

There is no wrong choice here, except maybe the choice of completely ignoring Yoga. The truth is that Yoga has been around for centuries and there's a reason why it has stayed alive for so long. It has been adopted by so many religions and cultures and has been adapted by so many people from around the world that it is now truly a global phenomenon.

With this book you got a glimpse into the Vedic life. I would recommend that you try to find out more about the Vedic society because it really had a lot of things figured out that we are still struggling with today. Now more than ever, the world can benefit from the Vedas and the way of life known as Yoga.

15700498R00030

Printed in Poland
by Amazon Fulfillment
Poland Sp. z o.o., Wrocław